MIGRAINE RELIEF PLAN AND COOKBOOK

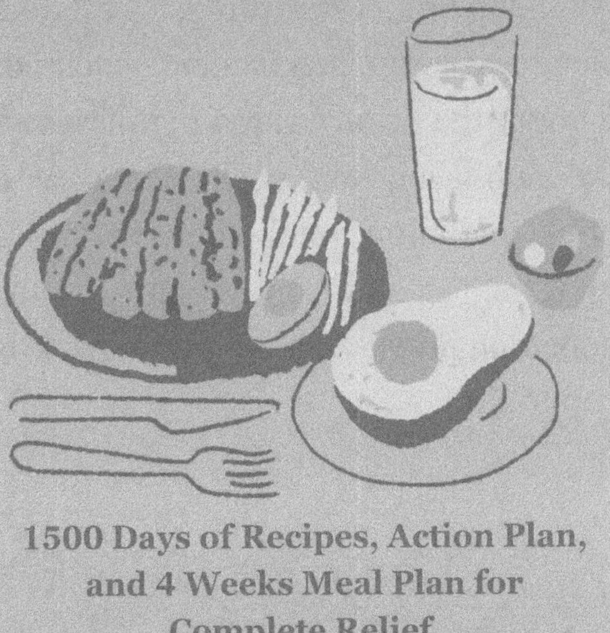

1500 Days of Recipes, Action Plan, and 4 Weeks Meal Plan for Complete Relief

Dr. Diane Reyes

Table of Contents

Introduction   **7**

    A. Understanding Migraines   9

    B. Importance of Lifestyle and Nutrition in Migraine Management   10

II. Migraine Basics   **14**

    A. Types of Migraines   14

    B. Triggers and Identifying Them   16

III. The Migraine Relief Plan   **19**

    A. Holistic Approaches   19

    B. Dietary Strategies   20

IV. Lifestyle Changes   **23**

    A. Exercise and its Impact   23

    B. Mindfulness and Relaxation Techniques 25

V. Managing Migraines in Different Situations   **28**

    A. Travelling   28

    B. Social Events   30

VI Recipes for Migraine Relief   **33**

A. Breakfast   **33**

    Avocado and Spinach Omelette   33

    Quinoa Breakfast Bowl   34

    Greek Yogurt Parfait   35

Banana Walnut Smoothie   36

Sweet Potato Toast with Almond Butter   37

Chia Pudding with Mango   38

Spinach and Feta Breakfast Wrap   39

Blueberry Almond Overnight Oats   40

Egg and Veggie Breakfast Muffins   41

Coconut and Berry Smoothie Bowl   42

Almond Flour Pancakes   43

Turmeric and Ginger Smoothie   44

Salmon and Avocado Toast   45

Berry and Almond Butter Smoothie   46

Pumpkin Chia Seed Pudding   47

Lunch Recipes   48

Quinoa and Chickpea Bowl   49

Greek Yogurt Chicken Wrap   50

Salmon and Quinoa Salad   51

Sweet Potato and Black Bean Bowl   52

Chickpea and Veggie Stir-Fry   53

Turkey and Avocado Wrap   54

Mango Chicken Quinoa Bowl   55

Vegetarian Lentil Soup   56

Caprese Quinoa Salad   57

Pesto Zucchini Noodles with Shrimp   58

Blackened Salmon Salad   59

Mediterranean Chickpea Salad   60

Turkey and Quinoa Stuffed Peppers   61

Vegetarian Buddha Bowl   62

Dinner Recipes   **63**

Avocado and Spinach Stuffed Chicken
Breast   63

Quinoa and Chickpea Stuffed Bell Peppers
64

Greek Yogurt Chicken Salad Wrap   65

Salmon and Quinoa Stuffed Zucchini   66

Sweet Potato and Black Bean Quesadillas:
67

Chickpea and Veggie Stir-Fry   68

Turkey and Avocado Lettuce Wraps   69

Mango Chicken Quinoa Bowl   70

Vegetarian Lentil Soup   71

Caprese Quinoa Salad   72

Pesto Zucchini Noodles with Shrimp   73

Blackened Salmon Salad   74

Mediterranean Chickpea Salad   75

Turkey and Quinoa Stuffed Peppers   76

Vegetarian Buddha Bowl   77

Snacks and Desserts   **78**

Avocado and Hummus Dip   78

Greek Yogurt Parfait with Berries   79

Almond Butter and Banana Smoothie   80

Cucumber and Tzatziki Bites   81

Dark Chocolate and Almond Clusters   82

Apple and Almond Butter Slices   83

Chia Seed Pudding with Berries   84

Frozen Grapes and Yogurt Popsicles   85

Coconut and Berry Smoothie Bowl 86

Trail Mix with Nuts and Dried Fruits 87

Cottage Cheese and Pineapple Bowl 88

Yogurt-Dipped Strawberries 89

Carrot and Hummus Sticks 90

Peach and Almond Yogurt Parfait 91

Chocolate Banana Bites 92

Beverages **93**

Ginger and Lemon Herbal Tea 93

Peppermint Iced Tea 94

Turmeric Golden Milk 95

Chamomile Lavender Tea 96

Berry and Spinach Smoothie 97

Cucumber and Mint Infused Water 98

Coconut Water Electrolyte Drink 99

Green Tea Citrus Refresher 100

Pineapple and Ginger Smoothie 101

Hibiscus Iced Tea 102

VII. 28 Days Migraine Relief Meal Plan **103**

Week 1 103

Week 2 106

Week 3 109

Week 4 112

IX. Conclusion **115**

A. Recap and Encouragement 115

B. Moving Forward with the Migraine Relief Plan 117

Introduction

In the quiet moments between the throbbing pain and the quest for relief, many have found themselves searching for a beacon of hope amid the labyrinth of migraines. It's a journey marked by frustration, resilience, and an unwavering desire to regain control over one's well-being. Imagine a world where that labyrinth is illuminated by a guiding light, offering not just solace but a comprehensive map leading to the sanctuary of relief. This is the promise of the "Migraine Relief Plan and Cookbook."

Let me share with you the story of Nancy, a resilient soul whose life was interwoven with the relentless rhythm of migraines. In the midst of her struggle, Nancy discovered a transformative path – a journey outlined in the pages of this book. As Nancy delved into the carefully crafted relief plan and savoured the nourishing recipes, she felt a shift. It was not just the recipes, but the holistic approach that unfolded, embracing stress management, dietary strategies, and mindfulness techniques. Each page resonated with the promise of a brighter dawn, free from the shadows of migraines.

Nancy's story is not unique, for it mirrors the countless narratives of those seeking refuge from the storm of migraines. As you embark on this journey with the "Migraine Relief Plan and Cookbook," let it be a beacon of hope, a testament that relief is not a distant dream but a tangible reality waiting to be embraced. The solution you've been seeking, the relief you've been yearning for – it's woven into the fabric of these pages, ready to unfold as you turn each one. Your journey towards a life unburdened by migraines begins here.

A. Understanding Migraines

Migraines are neurological disorders characterised by intense, throbbing headaches, often accompanied by nausea, vomiting, and sensitivity to light and sound. These episodes can last for hours to days, significantly impacting an individual's daily life. While the exact cause of migraines is not fully understood, a combination of genetic and environmental factors is believed to contribute.

Triggers for migraines vary among individuals and can include certain foods, hormonal changes, stress, lack of sleep, and environmental factors. The underlying mechanism involves abnormal brain activity affecting nerve signals, blood flow, and chemicals in the brain.

Treatment options range from medications targeting pain and symptoms to preventive measures addressing triggers and lifestyle modifications.

Identifying and managing triggers, along with a personalised treatment plan, are essential for effective migraine management.

B. Importance of Lifestyle and Nutrition in Migraine Management

Maintaining Regular Sleep Patterns:

Adequate and consistent sleep is crucial in managing migraines. Disruptions in sleep patterns can trigger attacks, so establishing a regular sleep routine can help reduce the frequency and severity of migraines.

Hydration:

Dehydration is a common migraine trigger. Maintaining proper hydration levels by drinking an adequate amount of water throughout the day can be beneficial in preventing attacks.

Balanced Nutrition:

Adopting a well-balanced diet can play a significant role in migraine management. Certain foods may act as triggers for some individuals, and identifying and avoiding these can be essential. Additionally, incorporating magnesium-rich foods, like nuts and leafy greens, may provide relief as magnesium deficiency is linked to migraines.

Caffeine Management:

While some people find relief from migraines through moderate caffeine intake, excessive consumption can trigger headaches. It's important to find the right balance and monitor how caffeine affects individual migraine patterns.

Stress Reduction Techniques:

Chronic stress is a common trigger for migraines. Incorporating stress-reduction techniques such as mindfulness, meditation, and yoga into daily life can contribute to better migraine management.

Regular Exercise:

Engaging in regular physical activity has been shown to reduce the frequency and intensity of migraines. However, it's important to maintain a consistent exercise routine and be mindful of individual limits to avoid triggering headaches.

Hormonal Balance:

For some individuals, hormonal changes, particularly in women during menstruation or menopause, can influence migraine patterns. Seeking guidance from healthcare professionals for hormonal management strategies may be beneficial.

A holistic approach to migraine management involves understanding individual triggers, adopting a healthy lifestyle, and maintaining a balanced diet. By incorporating these elements, individuals can gain better control over their migraines and improve their overall quality of life.

II. Migraine Basics

A. Types of Migraines

Migraine without Aura:

The most common type, characterised by moderate to severe pulsating headaches that can last from a few hours to several days. These headaches are often accompanied by symptoms such as nausea, vomiting, and sensitivity to light and sound.

Migraine with Aura:

In addition to the typical migraine symptoms, individuals may experience visual disturbances, such as flashing lights, blind spots, or tingling sensations. Aura usually occurs before the onset of the headache and can last up to an hour.

Chronic Migraines:

Defined by experiencing headaches on 15 or more days per month for at least three months, with at least eight of those headaches being migraines. Chronic migraines can significantly impact daily life and often require a comprehensive management plan.

Menstrual Migraines:

Occurring in relation to a woman's menstrual cycle, typically in the days leading up to or during menstruation. Hormonal fluctuations are believed to play a role in triggering these migraines.

Vestibular Migraines:

Associated with vertigo and issues related to balance and coordination. Individuals may experience dizziness, problems with spatial orientation, and difficulty with coordination during an episode.

B. Triggers and Identifying Them

Food Triggers:

Certain foods and beverages can act as triggers for migraines. Common culprits include aged cheeses, chocolate, caffeine, alcohol, and processed foods containing additives like monosodium glutamate (MSG). Keeping a food diary can help identify personal triggers.

Environmental Factors:

Sensitivity to light, noise, or strong odors can trigger migraines. Changes in weather, exposure to bright lights, and strong smells are common environmental triggers. Managing exposure to these factors can help reduce the frequency of migraines.

Hormonal Changes:

Fluctuations in oestrogen levels, especially in women during menstruation, pregnancy, or menopause, can trigger migraines. Understanding hormonal patterns and seeking medical advice for hormone-related management can be crucial.

Stress and Emotional Factors:

Emotional stress, anxiety, and tension are well-known triggers for migraines. Developing effective stress management techniques, such as mindfulness and relaxation exercises, can contribute to migraine prevention.

Sleep Patterns:

Irregular sleep patterns, insufficient sleep, or changes in sleep routine can trigger migraines. Establishing a consistent sleep schedule and practising good sleep hygiene are important steps in migraine management.

Physical Factors:

Intense physical exertion or sudden changes in physical activity levels can trigger migraines. Gradual adjustments to exercise routines and ensuring proper hydration are essential in preventing exercise-induced migraines.

Medication Overuse:

Ironically, the overuse of certain medications, including pain relievers, can lead to medication-overuse headaches, exacerbating migraine symptoms. It's crucial to follow healthcare provider guidelines for medication use.

Identifying and managing triggers is a key aspect of migraine management. Keeping a detailed record of migraine episodes, lifestyle factors, and potential triggers can aid healthcare professionals in developing personalised treatment plans for individuals suffering from migraines.

III. The Migraine Relief Plan

A. Holistic Approaches

Stress Management:

Stress is a common trigger for migraines, and adopting effective stress management techniques is crucial. Practices such as mindfulness meditation, deep breathing exercises, yoga, and progressive muscle relaxation can help reduce stress levels. Integrating these techniques into daily routines can contribute to overall well-being and migraine relief.

Sleep Hygiene:

Maintaining healthy sleep habits is vital in preventing migraines. Establishing a regular sleep schedule, creating a comfortable sleep environment, and practising relaxation techniques before bedtime can improve the quality and duration of sleep. Consistent, restful sleep contributes significantly to migraine relief.

B. Dietary Strategies

Migraine-Friendly Foods:

Certain foods are known to be migraine-friendly and can be included in a relief plan. These may include:

Magnesium-rich foods like nuts, seeds, and leafy greens.

Foods with omega-3 fatty acids, such as fatty fish (salmon, mackerel) and flaxseeds.

Ginger, known for its anti-inflammatory properties, may offer relief for some individuals.

Complex carbohydrates like whole grains, which provide a steady release of energy without causing spikes in blood sugar.

Meal Planning:

Structuring meals to prevent hunger-related triggers is essential. It's recommended to:

Eat regular, balanced meals to maintain stable blood sugar levels.

Avoid skipping meals, as this can lead to low blood sugar, triggering migraines.

Identify and eliminate potential trigger foods by keeping a detailed food diary.

Stay hydrated by drinking an adequate amount of water throughout the day.

Creating a meal plan that aligns with these principles can be a valuable component of a migraine relief strategy. Consulting with a healthcare professional or a registered dietitian to develop a personalised meal plan based on individual triggers and dietary needs is advisable.

A comprehensive migraine relief plan incorporates holistic approaches, including stress management and sleep hygiene, along with dietary strategies that focus on migraine-friendly foods and well-structured meal planning. Integrating these elements into daily life can contribute to reducing the frequency and severity of migraines, providing individuals with a proactive approach to managing their condition.

IV. Lifestyle Changes

A. Exercise and its Impact

Regular exercise is a crucial component of a healthy lifestyle and can have a positive impact on migraine management. Here's how:

Improved Blood Flow:

Exercise promotes better blood circulation, reducing the risk of vascular changes that can trigger migraines. It also helps maintain stable blood pressure, contributing to overall vascular health.

Stress Reduction:

Physical activity is a natural stress reliever. Engaging in regular exercise releases endorphins, the body's natural mood lifters, helping to alleviate stress and tension—common triggers for migraines.

Regulated Sleep Patterns:

Regular exercise can contribute to better sleep quality and duration. Establishing a consistent exercise routine helps regulate the body's internal clock, promoting more restful sleep and reducing the likelihood of sleep-related migraine triggers.

Weight Management:

Maintaining a healthy weight is essential for migraine management. Regular exercise, coupled with a balanced diet, contributes to weight control and reduces the risk of obesity-related migraines.

Tension Relief:

Many migraines are associated with muscle tension, especially in the neck and shoulders. Exercise helps alleviate tension, promoting relaxation and reducing the likelihood of tension-induced migraines.

It's important to note that individuals should choose exercises that suit their fitness level and preferences. Starting with low-impact activities and gradually increasing intensity can help prevent exercise-induced migraines.

B. Mindfulness and Relaxation Techniques

Meditation:

Mindfulness meditation involves focusing attention on the present moment without judgement. Regular meditation practice can reduce stress, improve emotional well-being, and contribute to overall migraine relief.

Deep Breathing Exercises:

Controlled breathing techniques, such as diaphragmatic breathing or paced breathing, can activate the body's relaxation response. These exercises help lower stress levels and promote a calm state of mind, potentially preventing stress-induced migraines.

Progressive Muscle Relaxation (PMR):

PMR involves systematically tensing and then relaxing different muscle groups in the body. This technique helps release physical tension, providing relief from muscle-related migraine triggers.

Yoga:

Combining physical postures, breath control, and mindfulness, yoga offers a holistic approach to relaxation. Regular practice can improve flexibility, reduce muscle tension, and enhance overall well-being.

Biofeedback:

Biofeedback involves using electronic monitoring to gain awareness and control over physiological processes. This technique can be helpful in identifying and managing physical responses to stress, potentially reducing the frequency of stress-related migraines.

Incorporating exercise and mindfulness practices into daily life can significantly contribute to a comprehensive lifestyle approach to migraine management. It's advisable to consult with healthcare professionals or specialists to tailor these lifestyle changes to individual needs and ensure a safe and effective migraine relief plan.

V. Managing Migraines in Different Situations

A. Travelling

Travelling can present unique challenges for individuals prone to migraines. Here are strategies to manage migraines during travel:

Plan Ahead:

Schedule travel during times when migraines are less likely to occur.

Plan for breaks during long journeys to rest and manage stress.

Stay Hydrated:

Dehydration is a common trigger, so ensure adequate water intake, especially during flights.

Limit caffeine and alcohol, as they can contribute to dehydration.

Protect Against Sensory Triggers:

Wear sunglasses to reduce sensitivity to bright lights.

Use noise-cancelling headphones or earplugs to minimise exposure to loud sounds.

Pack Medications:

Carry prescribed medications in your hand luggage.

Pack an emergency migraine kit with pain relievers, nausea medication, and any other prescribed items.

Manage Sleep Patterns:

Adjust to new time zones gradually to minimise disruptions to sleep patterns.

Use travel pillows and blankets to create a comfortable sleep environment during transit.

Mindful Eating:

Be mindful of food triggers, especially when trying new cuisines.

Plan meals to avoid skipping or delaying them, preventing hunger-induced migraines.

B. Social Events

Attending social events can be challenging when managing migraines. Consider the following tips:

Communicate Openly:

Inform close friends or event organisers about your condition so they can provide support if needed.

Communicate any dietary restrictions or preferences to ensure migraine-friendly food options.

Choose Well-Lit Spaces:

Opt for well-lit environments to minimise sensitivity to lighting.

Position yourself away from strobe lights or flashing decorations.

Manage Noise Levels:

Choose quieter areas during events to reduce exposure to loud music or conversations.

Bring earplugs to use when needed.

Prioritize Self-Care:

Allow yourself breaks to rest and relax, especially if the event is lengthy.

Avoid overcommitting to multiple social events in a short period.

Plan Transportation:

Arrange reliable transportation to and from the event to minimise stress.

Ensure there's a quiet and comfortable space available if transportation involves long periods.

Prepare an Emergency Kit:

Carry a small bag with essential migraine relief items, including medication, water, and any comfort items.

Create a Support System:

Attend events with understanding friends or family who can provide assistance if a migraine occurs.

Establish a discrete signal or communication method with someone you trust.

Adapting these strategies to personal preferences and triggers can enhance the ability to manage migraines effectively in various situations. Flexibility and preparation are key when navigating travel or social events while dealing with migraines.

VI Recipes for Migraine Relief

A. Breakfast

Avocado and Spinach Omelette

Ingredients:

2 eggs

1/2 avocado, sliced

Handful of spinach

Instructions:

Whisk eggs in a bowl.

Heat a pan and pour whisked eggs.

Add sliced avocado and spinach to one side.

Get the omelette folded and cook until eggs are set.

Nutritional Value (approx.):Calories: 300

Protein: 15g

Fat: 20g

Carbohydrates: 12g

Quinoa Breakfast Bowl

Ingredients:

1/2 cup cooked quinoa

1/4 cup almond milk

1 tablespoon chia seeds

Fresh berries

Instructions:

Mix quinoa, almond milk, and chia seeds in a bowl.

Top with fresh berries.

Nutritional Value (approx.):

Calories: 250

Protein: 8g

Fat: 6g

Carbohydrates: 40g

Greek Yogurt Parfait

Ingredients:

1 cup Greek yogurt

1/2 cup granola

1/4 cup mixed berries

Instructions:

Get Greek yogurt, granola, and mixed berries layered in a glass or bowl.

Nutritional Value (approx.):

Calories: 300

Protein: 15g

Fat: 8g

Carbohydrates: 40g

Banana Walnut Smoothie

Ingredients:

1 ripe banana

1/4 cup walnuts

1 cup almond milk

Instructions:

Blend banana, walnuts, and almond milk until smooth.

Nutritional Value (approx.):

Calories: 350

Protein: 7g

Fat: 18g

Carbohydrates: 45g

Sweet Potato Toast with Almond Butter

Ingredients:

1 sweet potato, sliced and toasted

2 tablespoons almond butter

Instructions:

Toast sweet potato slices.

Spread almond butter on the toasted sweet potato.

Nutritional Value (approx.):

Calories: 200

Protein: 5g

Fat: 12g

Carbohydrates: 22g

Chia Pudding with Mango

Ingredients:

2 tablespoons chia seeds

1/2 cup coconut milk

Fresh mango slices

Instructions:

Get chia seeds and coconut milk mixed in a jar.

Refrigerate overnight.

Top with fresh mango slices before serving.

Nutritional Value (approx.):

Calories: 250

Protein: 5g

Fat: 15g

Carbohydrates: 30g

Spinach and Feta Breakfast Wrap

Ingredients:

1 whole-grain tortilla

Handful of fresh spinach

2 tablespoons feta cheese

Instructions:

Place fresh spinach on the tortilla.

Sprinkle feta cheese over the spinach.

Fold into a wrap.

Nutritional Value (approx.):

Calories: 300

Protein: 12g

Fat: 15g

Carbohydrates: 30g

Blueberry Almond Overnight Oats

Ingredients:

1/2 cup rolled oats

1/2 cup almond milk

1/4 cup blueberries

1 tablespoon almond slices

Instructions:

Combine rolled oats and almond milk in a jar.

Mix in blueberries and refrigerate overnight.

Top with almond slices before serving.

Nutritional Value (approx.):

Calories: 280

Protein: 7g

Fat: 10g

Carbohydrates: 40g

Egg and Veggie Breakfast Muffins

Ingredients:

4 eggs

Chopped veggies (bell peppers, tomatoes, spinach)

Instructions:

Preheat the oven to 350°F (175°C).

Whisk eggs in a bowl.

Stir in chopped veggies.

Pour the mixture into greased muffin cups.

Let them bake for 15-20 minutes or until eggs are set.

Nutritional Value (approx.): Calories: 200

Protein: 14g

Fat: 12g

Carbohydrates: 10g

Coconut and Berry Smoothie Bowl

Ingredients:

1/2 cup coconut water

1/2 cup mixed berries

1/4 cup shredded coconut

Instructions:

Blend coconut water and mixed berries until smooth.

Pour the smoothie into a bowl.

Top with shredded coconut.

Nutritional Value (approx.):

Calories: 220

Protein: 3g

Fat: 8g

Carbohydrates: 35g

Almond Flour Pancakes

Ingredients:

1 cup almond flour

2 eggs

1/2 cup almond milk

Instructions:

In a bowl, mix almond flour, eggs, and almond milk until well combined.

Heat a griddle or pan over moderate heat.

Onto the griddle, spoon the batter to form pancakes.

Cook until bubbles emerges on the surface, then flip and cook the other part.

Nutritional Value (approx.): Calories: 280

Protein: 12g Fat: 20g

Carbohydrates: 10g

Turmeric and Ginger Smoothie

Ingredients:

1 cup coconut milk

1/2 teaspoon turmeric

1/2 teaspoon grated ginger

1/2 banana

Instructions:

Blend coconut milk, turmeric, grated ginger, and banana until smooth.

Pour into a glass and enjoy.

Nutritional Value (approx.):

Calories: 220

Protein: 2g

Fat: 15g

Carbohydrates: 25g

Salmon and Avocado Toast

Ingredients:

2 slices whole-grain bread

Smoked salmon

1/2 avocado, mashed

Instructions:

Toast slices of whole-grain bread.

Spread mashed avocado evenly on the toast.

Top with smoked salmon.

Nutritional Value (approx.):

Calories: 300

Protein: 15g

Fat: 15g

Carbohydrates: 25g

Berry and Almond Butter Smoothie

Ingredients:

1 cup mixed berries (strawberries, blueberries, raspberries)

1 tablespoon almond butter

1/2 cup Greek yogurt

Instructions:

Blend mixed berries, almond butter, and Greek yogurt until smooth.

Pour into a glass and enjoy.

Nutritional Value (approx.):

Calories: 280

Protein: 10g

Fat: 14g

Carbohydrates: 30g

Pumpkin Chia Seed Pudding

Ingredients:

1/2 cup canned pumpkin puree

2 tablespoons chia seeds

1/2 teaspoon cinnamon

1/2 cup almond milk

Instructions:

In a bowl, mix pumpkin puree, chia seeds, cinnamon, and almond milk.

Refrigerate for a minimum of two hours or overnight.

Stir well before serving.

Nutritional Value (approx.):

Calories: 180

Protein: 4g

Fat: 10g Carbohydrates: 20g

Lunch Recipes

Avocado and Spinach Salad with Grilled Chicken

Ingredients:

2 cups fresh spinach

1/2 avocado, sliced

Grilled chicken breast slices

Instructions:

Combine fresh spinach and avocado in a bowl.

Top with grilled chicken breast slices.

Nutritional Value (approx.):

Calories: 350

Protein: 30g

Fat: 18g

Carbohydrates: 15g

Quinoa and Chickpea Bowl

Ingredients:

1 cup cooked quinoa

1/2 cup chickpeas, drained

Mixed vegetables (bell peppers, cucumber, cherry tomatoes)

Instructions:

Combine cooked quinoa, chickpeas, and mixed vegetables in a bowl.

Nutritional Value (approx.):

Calories: 300

Protein: 12g

Fat: 8g

Carbohydrates: 45g

Greek Yogurt Chicken Wrap

Ingredients:

Grilled chicken strips

Whole-grain tortilla

1/2 cup Greek yogurt

Chopped tomatoes and cucumbers

Instructions:

Spread Greek yogurt on a whole-grain tortilla.

Add grilled chicken, chopped tomatoes, and cucumbers.

Wrap it up and enjoy.

Nutritional Value (approx.): Calories: 380

Protein: 25g

Fat: 15g

Carbohydrates: 40g

Salmon and Quinoa Salad

Ingredients:

Grilled salmon fillet

1 cup cooked quinoa

Mixed greens (arugula, spinach)

Lemon vinaigrette dressing

Instructions:

Place grilled salmon on a bed of mixed greens and quinoa.

Drizzle with lemon vinaigrette.

Nutritional Value (approx.):

Calories: 400

Protein: 30g

Fat: 20g

Carbohydrates: 25g

Sweet Potato and Black Bean Bowl

Ingredients:

Roasted sweet potato cubes

1/2 cup black beans, drained

Sliced avocado

Instructions:

Combine roasted sweet potato, black beans, and sliced avocado.

Nutritional Value (approx.):

Calories: 320

Protein: 10g

Fat: 15g

Carbohydrates: 40g

Chickpea and Veggie Stir-Fry

Ingredients:

1 cup chickpeas, cooked

Mixed vegetables (broccoli, bell peppers, snap peas)

Quinoa or brown rice

Instructions:

Stir-fry mixed vegetables and chickpeas in a pan.

Enjoy over either a bed of quinoa or brown rice.

Nutritional Value (approx.):

Calories: 380

Protein: 15g

Fat: 10g

Carbohydrates: 55g

Turkey and Avocado Wrap

Ingredients:

Sliced turkey breast

Whole-grain wrap

1/2 avocado, sliced

Lettuce and tomato

Instructions:

Layer sliced turkey, avocado, lettuce, and tomato on a whole-grain wrap.

Roll it up and enjoy.

Nutritional Value (approx.):

Calories: 320

Protein: 25g

Fat: 15g

Carbohydrates: 30g

Mango Chicken Quinoa Bowl

Ingredients:

Grilled chicken breast

1/2 cup cooked quinoa

Mango slices

Mixed greens

Instructions:

Arrange grilled chicken, cooked quinoa, mango slices, and mixed greens in a bowl.

Nutritional Value (approx.):

Calories: 350

Protein: 30g

Fat: 10g

Carbohydrates: 40g

Vegetarian Lentil Soup

Ingredients:

1 cup lentils, rinsed

Mixed vegetables (carrots, celery, onion)

Vegetable broth

Instructions:

Cook lentils and mixed vegetables in vegetable broth until tender.

Season to taste and enjoy.

Nutritional Value (approx.):

Calories: 280

Protein: 15g

Fat: 5g

Carbohydrates: 45g

Caprese Quinoa Salad

Ingredients:

1 cup cooked quinoa

Cherry tomatoes, halved

Fresh mozzarella, diced

Fresh basil leaves

Instructions:

Mix cooked quinoa, cherry tomatoes, fresh mozzarella, and basil.

Drizzle with balsamic glaze.

Nutritional Value (approx.):

Calories: 320

Protein: 15g

Fat: 15g

Carbohydrates: 30g

Pesto Zucchini Noodles with Shrimp

Ingredients:

Zucchini noodles

Shrimp, peeled and deveined

Pesto sauce

Cherry tomatoes

Instructions:

Saute shrimp in a pan until cooked.

Toss zucchini noodles, shrimp, pesto sauce, and cherry tomatoes.

Nutritional Value (approx.):

Calories: 300

Protein: 25g

Fat: 15g

Carbohydrates: 20g

Blackened Salmon Salad

Ingredients:

Blackened salmon fillet

Mixed greens

Cucumber slices

Balsamic vinaigrette

Instructions:

Place blackened salmon on a bed of mixed greens.

Add cucumber slices and drizzle with balsamic vinaigrette.

Nutritional Value (approx.):

Calories: 350

Protein: 30g

Fat: 18g

Carbohydrates: 15g

Mediterranean Chickpea Salad

Ingredients:

1 cup chickpeas, cooked

Cherry tomatoes, halved

Cucumber, diced

Feta cheese, crumbled

Instructions:

Get the chickpeas, cherry tomatoes, cucumber, and feta cheese mixed.

Drizzle with olive oil and season to taste.

Nutritional Value (approx.):

Calories: 280

Protein: 14g

Fat: 15g

Carbohydrates: 30g

Turkey and Quinoa Stuffed Peppers

Ingredients:

Ground turkey

Cooked quinoa

Bell peppers, halved

Tomato sauce

Instructions:

Brown ground turkey, mix with cooked quinoa.

Stuff bell peppers with the turkey and quinoa mixture.

Bake until peppers are tender.

Nutritional Value (approx.): Calories: 320

Protein: 25g

Fat: 12g

Carbohydrates: 30g

Vegetarian Buddha Bowl

Ingredients:

Brown rice

Roasted sweet potato

Sauteed kale

Hummus

Instructions:

Arrange brown rice, roasted sweet potato, and sauteed kale in a bowl.

Top with a dollop of hummus.

Nutritional Value (approx.):

Calories: 350

Protein: 10g

Fat: 10g

Carbohydrates: 55g

Dinner Recipes

Avocado and Spinach Stuffed Chicken Breast

Ingredients:

Chicken breast

1/2 avocado, mashed

Handful of fresh spinach

Instructions:

Preheat oven to 375°F (190°C).

Cut a pocket into the chicken breast.

Stuff with mashed avocado and fresh spinach.

Bake until chicken is cooked through.

Nutritional Value (approx.): Calories: 400

Protein: 35g Fat: 20g

Carbohydrates: 15g

Quinoa and Chickpea Stuffed Bell Peppers

Ingredients:

Bell peppers, halved

1 cup cooked quinoa

1/2 cup chickpeas, drained

Diced tomatoes and onions

Instructions:

Preheat oven to 375°F (190°C).

Mix quinoa, chickpeas, diced tomatoes, and onions.

Stuff bell peppers and bake until peppers are tender.

Nutritional Value (approx.): Calories: 350

Protein: 15g Fat: 10g

Carbohydrates: 50g

Greek Yogurt Chicken Salad Wrap

Ingredients:

Grilled chicken strips

Whole-grain wrap

1/2 cup Greek yogurt

Chopped cucumbers and cherry tomatoes

Instructions:

Mix grilled chicken, Greek yogurt, cucumbers, and cherry tomatoes.

Spread the mixture on a whole-grain wrap and roll it up.

Nutritional Value (approx.):

Calories: 380

Protein: 30g

Fat: 15g

Carbohydrates: 35g

Salmon and Quinoa Stuffed Zucchini

Ingredients:

Zucchini, halved

Grilled salmon flakes

1 cup cooked quinoa

Dill and lemon for garnish

Instructions:

Preheat oven to 375°F (190°C).

Scoop out zucchini centers and stuff with a mixture of grilled salmon and quinoa.

Bake until zucchini is tender.

Nutritional Value (approx.): Calories: 380

Protein: 30g

Fat: 18g

Carbohydrates: 25g

Sweet Potato and Black Bean Quesadillas:

Ingredients:

Sweet potato, mashed

Black beans, mashed

Whole-grain tortillas

Avocado slices

Instructions:

Spread mashed sweet potato and black beans on a tortilla.

Top with avocado slices and fold in half.

Nutritional Value (approx.):

Calories: 320

Protein: 10g

Fat: 15g

Carbohydrates: 40g

Chickpea and Veggie Stir-Fry

Ingredients:

1 cup chickpeas, cooked

Mixed vegetables (broccoli, bell peppers, snap peas)

Quinoa or brown rice

Instructions:

Stir-fry mixed vegetables and chickpeas in a pan.

Enjoy over either a bed of quinoa or brown rice.

Nutritional Value (approx.):

Calories: 380

Protein: 15g

Fat: 10g

Carbohydrates: 55g

Turkey and Avocado Lettuce Wraps

Ingredients:

Ground turkey

Lettuce leaves

1/2 avocado, sliced

Salsa for topping

Instructions:

Cook ground turkey and season to taste.

Spoon turkey into lettuce leaves, top with sliced avocado and salsa.

Nutritional Value (approx.):

Calories: 320

Protein: 25g

Fat: 15g

Carbohydrates: 20g

Mango Chicken Quinoa Bowl

Ingredients:

Grilled chicken breast

1/2 cup cooked quinoa

Mango slices

Mixed greens

Instructions:

Arrange grilled chicken, cooked quinoa, mango slices, and mixed greens in a bowl.

Nutritional Value (approx.):

Calories: 350

Protein: 30g

Fat: 10g

Carbohydrates: 40g

Vegetarian Lentil Soup

Ingredients:

1 cup lentils, rinsed

Mixed vegetables (carrots, celery, onion)

Vegetable broth

Instructions:

Cook lentils and mixed vegetables in vegetable broth until tender.

Season to taste and enjoy.

Nutritional Value (approx.):

Calories: 280

Protein: 15g

Fat: 5g

Carbohydrates: 45g

Caprese Quinoa Salad

Ingredients:

1 cup cooked quinoa

Cherry tomatoes, halved

Fresh mozzarella, diced

Fresh basil leaves

Instructions:

Mix cooked quinoa, cherry tomatoes, fresh mozzarella, and basil.

Drizzle with balsamic glaze.

Nutritional Value (approx.):

Calories: 320

Protein: 15g

Fat: 15g

Carbohydrates: 30g

Pesto Zucchini Noodles with Shrimp

Ingredients:

Zucchini noodles

Shrimp, peeled and deveined

Pesto sauce

Cherry tomatoes

Instructions:

Saute shrimp in a pan until cooked.

Toss zucchini noodles, shrimp, pesto sauce, and cherry tomatoes.

Nutritional Value (approx.):

Calories: 300

Protein: 25g

Fat: 15g

Carbohydrates: 20g

Blackened Salmon Salad

Ingredients:

Blackened salmon fillet

Mixed greens

Cucumber slices

Balsamic vinaigrette

Instructions:

Place blackened salmon on a bed of mixed greens.

Add cucumber slices and drizzle with balsamic vinaigrette.

Nutritional Value (approx.):

Calories: 350

Protein: 30g

Fat: 18g

Carbohydrates: 15g

Mediterranean Chickpea Salad

Ingredients:

1 cup chickpeas, cooked

Cherry tomatoes, halved

Cucumber, diced

Feta cheese, crumbled

Instructions:

Get the chickpeas, cherry tomatoes, cucumber, and feta cheese mixed.

Drizzle with olive oil and season to taste.

Nutritional Value (approx.):

Calories: 280

Protein: 14g

Fat: 15g

Carbohydrates: 30g

Turkey and Quinoa Stuffed Peppers

Ingredients:

Ground turkey

Cooked quinoa

Bell peppers, halved

Tomato sauce

Instructions:

Brown ground turkey, mix with cooked quinoa.

Stuff bell peppers with the turkey and quinoa mixture.

Bake until peppers are tender.

Nutritional Value (approx.): Calories: 320

Protein: 25g

Fat: 12g

Carbohydrates: 30g

Vegetarian Buddha Bowl

Ingredients:

Brown rice

Roasted sweet potato

Sauteed kale

Hummus

Instructions:

Arrange brown rice, roasted sweet potato, and sauteed kale in a bowl.

Top with a dollop of hummus.

Nutritional Value (approx.):

Calories: 350

Protein: 10g

Fat: 10g

Carbohydrates: 55g

Snacks and Desserts

Avocado and Hummus Dip

Ingredients:

1 ripe avocado, mashed

1/2 cup hummus

Baby carrots or cucumber slices for dipping

Instructions:

Mix mashed avocado with hummus.

Serve with baby carrots or cucumber slices.

Nutritional Value (approx.):

Calories: 180

Protein: 5g

Fat: 12g

Carbohydrates: 15g

Greek Yogurt Parfait with Berries

Ingredients:

1 cup Greek yogurt

Mixed berries (strawberries, blueberries, raspberries)

Granola

Instructions:

Layer Greek yogurt, mixed berries, and granola in a glass or bowl.

Nutritional Value (approx.):

Calories: 250

Protein: 15g

Fat: 8g

Carbohydrates: 35g

Almond Butter and Banana Smoothie

Ingredients:

1 banana

2 tablespoons almond butter

1 cup almond milk

Instructions:

Blend banana, almond butter, and almond milk until smooth.

Nutritional Value (approx.):

Calories: 300

Protein: 7g

Fat: 18g

Carbohydrates: 35g

Cucumber and Tzatziki Bites

Ingredients:

Cucumber slices

Tzatziki sauce

Dill for garnish

Instructions:

Top cucumber slices with tzatziki sauce.

Garnish with dill.

Nutritional Value (approx.):

Calories: 120

Protein: 3g

Fat: 8g

Carbohydrates: 10g

Dark Chocolate and Almond Clusters

Ingredients:

Dark chocolate squares

Almonds

Instructions:

Melt dark chocolate and mix with almonds.

Spoon clusters onto parchment paper and let them cool.

Nutritional Value (approx. per cluster):

Calories: 50

Protein: 1g

Fat: 4g

Carbohydrates: 5g

Apple and Almond Butter Slices

Ingredients:

Apple slices

Almond butter

Instructions:

Spread almond butter on apple slices.

Nutritional Value (approx. per serving):

Calories: 150

Protein: 3g

Fat: 8g

Carbohydrates: 18g

Chia Seed Pudding with Berries

Ingredients:

2 tablespoons chia seeds

1 cup almond milk

Mixed berries

Instructions:

Mix chia seeds and almond milk, refrigerate until pudding-like consistency.

Top with mixed berries before serving.

Nutritional Value (approx.):

Calories: 200

Protein: 5g

Fat: 10g

Carbohydrates: 25g

Frozen Grapes and Yogurt Popsicles

Ingredients:

Red or green grapes

Greek yogurt

Instructions:

Dip grapes in Greek yogurt and freeze on a stick.

Nutritional Value (approx. per popsicle):

Calories: 80

Protein: 3g

Fat: 2g

Carbohydrates: 15g

Coconut and Berry Smoothie Bowl

Ingredients:

1/2 cup coconut water

Mixed berries

1/4 cup shredded coconut

Instructions:

Get the coconut water and mixed berries blended until smooth.

Pour into a bowl and top with shredded coconut.

Nutritional Value (approx.):

Calories: 220

Protein: 3g

Fat: 8g

Carbohydrates: 35g

Trail Mix with Nuts and Dried Fruits

Ingredients:

Almonds, walnuts, dried cranberries, and apricots

Instructions:

Mix almonds, walnuts, dried cranberries, and apricots in a bowl.

Nutritional Value (approx. per serving):

Calories: 200

Protein: 5g

Fat: 12g

Carbohydrates: 20g

Cottage Cheese and Pineapple Bowl

Ingredients:

Cottage cheese

Fresh pineapple chunks

Instructions:

Combine cottage cheese and fresh pineapple chunks in a bowl.

Nutritional Value (approx. per serving):

Calories: 180

Protein: 15g

Fat: 5g

Carbohydrates: 20g

Yogurt-Dipped Strawberries

Ingredients:

Fresh strawberries

Greek yogurt

Instructions:

Dip strawberries in Greek yogurt.

Place on a tray and freeze for a refreshing treat.

Nutritional Value (approx. per serving):

Calories: 120

Protein: 6g

Fat: 3g

Carbohydrates: 20g

Carrot and Hummus Sticks

Ingredients:

Carrot sticks

Hummus

Instructions:

Dip carrot sticks in hummus for a crunchy snack.

Nutritional Value (approx. per serving):

Calories: 100

Protein: 3g

Fat: 7g

Carbohydrates: 10g

Peach and Almond Yogurt Parfait

Ingredients:

Greek yogurt

Sliced peaches

Almond slices

Instructions:

Layer Greek yogurt, sliced peaches, and almond slices in a glass.

Nutritional Value (approx. per serving):

Calories: 220

Protein: 15g

Fat: 10g

Carbohydrates: 20g

Chocolate Banana Bites

Ingredients:

Banana slices

Dark chocolate

Chopped nuts (almonds, walnuts)

Instructions:

Dip banana slices in melted dark chocolate.

Sprinkle with chopped nuts and let them set.

Nutritional Value (approx. per serving):

Calories: 150

Protein: 3g

Fat: 8g

Carbohydrates: 20g

Beverages

Ginger and Lemon Herbal Tea

Ingredients:

Fresh ginger slices

Lemon juice

Honey (optional)

Instructions:

Steep fresh ginger slices in hot water.

Include a squeeze of lemon juice and honey to taste.

Benefits:

Ginger may help reduce nausea associated with migraines.

Lemon provides a refreshing flavor.

Peppermint Iced Tea

Ingredients:

Peppermint tea bags

Ice cubes

Fresh mint leaves (optional)

Instructions:

Brew peppermint tea and let it cool.

Pour over ice and garnish with fresh mint leaves.

Benefits:

Peppermint may have a calming effect on headaches.

Turmeric Golden Milk

Ingredients:

1 cup almond milk

1/2 teaspoon turmeric

Pinch of black pepper

Honey (optional)

Instructions:

Heat almond milk with turmeric and black pepper.

Sweeten with honey if desired.

Benefits:

Turmeric has anti-inflammatory properties.

Chamomile Lavender Tea

Ingredients:

Chamomile tea bags

Dried lavender (optional)

Honey (optional)

Instructions:

Brew chamomile tea and add dried lavender.

Sweeten with honey if desired.

Benefits:

Chamomile may have calming effects.

Berry and Spinach Smoothie

Ingredients:

Mixed berries (strawberries, blueberries)

Spinach leaves

Coconut water

Instructions:

Blend berries, spinach, and coconut water until smooth.

Benefits:

Berries provide antioxidants, and spinach offers nutrients.

Cucumber and Mint Infused Water

Ingredients:

Cucumber slices

Fresh mint leaves

Water

Instructions:

To the water, add cucumber slices and mint leaves

Let it infuse in the refrigerator for a refreshing drink.

Benefits:

Hydration is key for migraine relief.

Coconut Water Electrolyte Drink

Ingredients:

Coconut water

Splash of lime juice

Pinch of sea salt

Instructions:

Mix coconut water with lime juice and a pinch of sea salt.

Benefits:

Coconut water provides hydration and electrolytes.

Green Tea Citrus Refresher

Ingredients:

Green tea bags

Orange slices

Fresh lime juice

Instructions:

Brew green tea and let it cool.

Add orange slices and fresh lime juice.

Benefits:

Green tea contains antioxidants, and citrus adds a zesty twist.

Pineapple and Ginger Smoothie

Ingredients:

Fresh pineapple chunks

Ginger

Almond milk

Instructions:

Blend pineapple, ginger, and almond milk until smooth.

Benefits:

Pineapple provides natural sweetness, and ginger aids digestion.

Hibiscus Iced Tea

Ingredients:

Hibiscus tea bags

Ice cubes

Orange slices for garnish

Instructions:

Brew hibiscus tea and let it cool.

Serve over ice with orange slices.

Benefits:

Hibiscus tea may help lower blood pressure and provide hydration.

VII. 28 Days Migraine Relief Meal Plan

Week 1

Day 1:

Breakfast: Quinoa Porridge with Mixed Berries

Lunch: Chickpea and Veggie Stir-Fry over Brown Rice

Dinner: Avocado and Spinach Stuffed Chicken Breast

Day 2:

Breakfast: Greek Yogurt Parfait with Berries

Lunch: Turkey and Avocado Lettuce Wraps

Dinner: Quinoa and Chickpea Stuffed Bell Peppers

Day 3:

Breakfast: Almond Butter and Banana Smoothie

Lunch: Salmon and Quinoa Stuffed Zucchini

Dinner: Greek Yogurt Chicken Salad Wrap

Day 4:

Breakfast: Cottage Cheese and Pineapple Bowl

Lunch: Pesto Zucchini Noodles with Shrimp

Dinner: Vegetarian Buddha Bowl

Day 5:

Breakfast: Dark Chocolate and Almond Clusters

Lunch: Blackened Salmon Salad

Dinner: Mango Chicken Quinoa Bowl

Day 6:

Breakfast: Apple and Almond Butter Slices

Lunch: Mediterranean Chickpea Salad

Dinner: Turkey and Quinoa Stuffed Peppers

Day 7:

Breakfast: Chia Seed Pudding with Berries

Lunch: Caprese Quinoa Salad

Dinner: Vegetarian Lentil Soup

Week 2

Day 8:

Breakfast: Peach and Almond Yogurt Parfait

Lunch: Chickpea and Veggie Stir-Fry over Brown Rice

Dinner: Avocado and Spinach Stuffed Chicken Breast

Day 9:

Breakfast: Chocolate Banana Bites

Lunch: Turkey and Avocado Lettuce Wraps

Dinner: Quinoa and Chickpea Stuffed Bell Peppers

Day 10:

Breakfast: Cucumber and Mint Infused Water

Lunch: Salmon and Quinoa Stuffed Zucchini

Dinner: Greek Yogurt Chicken Salad Wrap

Day 11:

Breakfast: Yogurt-Dipped Strawberries

Lunch: Pesto Zucchini Noodles with Shrimp

Dinner: Vegetarian Buddha Bowl

Day 12:

Breakfast: Coconut Water Electrolyte Drink

Lunch: Blackened Salmon Salad

Dinner: Mango Chicken Quinoa Bowl

Day 13:

Breakfast: Carrot and Hummus Sticks

Lunch: Mediterranean Chickpea Salad

Dinner: Turkey and Quinoa Stuffed Peppers

Day 14:

Breakfast: Green Tea Citrus Refresher

Lunch: Caprese Quinoa Salad

Dinner: Vegetarian Lentil Soup

Week 3

Day 15:

Breakfast: Coconut and Berry Smoothie Bowl

Lunch: Chickpea and Veggie Stir-Fry over Brown Rice

Dinner: Avocado and Spinach Stuffed Chicken Breast

Day 16:

Breakfast: Almond Butter and Banana Smoothie

Lunch: Turkey and Avocado Lettuce Wraps

Dinner: Quinoa and Chickpea Stuffed Bell Peppers

Day 17:

Breakfast: Trail Mix with Nuts and Dried Fruits

Lunch: Salmon and Quinoa Stuffed Zucchini

Dinner: Greek Yogurt Chicken Salad Wrap

Day 18:

Breakfast: Chia Seed Pudding with Berries

Lunch: Pesto Zucchini Noodles with Shrimp

Dinner: Vegetarian Buddha Bowl

Day 19:

Breakfast: Frozen Grapes and Yogurt Popsicles

Lunch: Blackened Salmon Salad

Dinner: Mango Chicken Quinoa Bowl

Day 20:

Breakfast: Carrot and Hummus Sticks

Lunch: Mediterranean Chickpea Salad

Dinner: Turkey and Quinoa Stuffed Peppers

Day 21:

Breakfast: Pineapple and Ginger Smoothie

Lunch: Caprese Quinoa Salad

Dinner: Vegetarian Lentil Soup

Week 4

Day 22:

Breakfast: Apple and Almond Butter Slices

Lunch: Chickpea and Veggie Stir-Fry over Brown Rice

Dinner: Avocado and Spinach Stuffed Chicken Breast

Day 23:

Breakfast: Greek Yogurt Parfait with Berries

Lunch: Turkey and Avocado Lettuce Wraps

Dinner: Quinoa and Chickpea Stuffed Bell Peppers

Day 24:

Breakfast: Almond Butter and Banana Smoothie

Lunch: Salmon and Quinoa Stuffed Zucchini

Dinner: Greek Yogurt Chicken Salad Wrap

Day 25:

Breakfast: Cottage Cheese and Pineapple Bowl

Lunch: Pesto Zucchini Noodles with Shrimp

Dinner: Vegetarian Buddha Bowl

Day 26:

Breakfast: Dark Chocolate and Almond Clusters

Lunch: Blackened Salmon Salad

Dinner: Mango Chicken Quinoa Bowl

Day 27:

Breakfast: Apple and Almond Butter Slices

Lunch: Mediterranean Chickpea Salad

Dinner: Turkey and Quinoa Stuffed Peppers

Day 28:

Breakfast: Chia Seed Pudding with Berries

Lunch: Caprese Quinoa Salad

Dinner: Vegetarian Lentil Soup

IX. Conclusion

A. Recap and Encouragement

As we bring this transformative journey to a close, let's take a moment to reflect on the strides we've made and the path that lies ahead. The "Migraine Relief Plan and Cookbook" has not merely been a guide; it has been a companion on your quest for a life unshackled by the chains of migraines.

In this comprehensive journey, we've delved into the intricacies of migraines, uncovered the types, identified triggers, and harnessed the power of a holistic approach to relief. From stress management and sleep hygiene to carefully curated dietary strategies, each aspect has been meticulously woven into a tapestry of well-being. The recipes presented are not just nourishing for the body but a testament to the richness that life can offer when we take control of our health.

In moments of frustration, you discovered solace in the pages of shared stories and relatable experiences. Through the ups and downs, you've embraced the importance of lifestyle changes, learned to navigate migraines in different situations, and, above all, found a community within the pages of this guide – a community fueled by resilience and hope.

As you stand at the crossroads of your journey, take a moment to celebrate the progress you've made. The smallest steps are often the most significant, and your commitment to this path is commendable. You are not alone, and your pursuit of relief is a testament to your strength.

B. Moving Forward with the Migraine Relief Plan

Armed with the knowledge, strategies, and recipes encapsulated in the "Migraine Relief Plan and Cookbook," you now have the tools to forge ahead with confidence. Embrace the coming days as an opportunity to weave these practices into the fabric of your life. Consistency is the key, and each small adjustment you make contributes to the overarching narrative of your well-being.

Remember, the journey toward migraine relief is unique for each individual. Your path may have its twists and turns, but with the foundation laid in these pages, you possess the resilience to navigate them. Continue to prioritise self-care, stay attuned to your body's signals, and celebrate the victories – no matter how small.

This is not just an ending but a commencement – a launch into a future where migraines need not dictate the terms of your life. As you move forward, carry the learnings, the support, and the hope encapsulated in this guide. May your days be marked by vitality, and may the shadows of migraines dissipate in the radiant light of your well-being.

Your journey continues, and the "Migraine Relief Plan and Cookbook" remains a steadfast companion, ready to support you on the road ahead. May it be a source of inspiration, guidance, and, above all, the catalyst for a life free from the constraints of migraines.